Russell Thacher Trall

Water-Cure for the Million

The processes of water-cure explained: popular errors exposed; hygienic

and drug-medication contrasted; rules for bathing, dieting, exercising,

etc.; recipes for cooking; directions for home-treatment

Russell Thacher Trall

Water-Cure for the Million
*The processes of water-cure explained: popular errors exposed; hygienic and
drug-medication contrasted; rules for bathing, dieting, exercising, etc.; recipes for
cooking; directions for home-treatment*

ISBN/EAN: 9783337102227

Printed in Europe, USA, Canada, Australia, Japan

Cover: Foto ©Lupo / pixelio.de

More available books at **www.hansebooks.com**

WATER-CURE

FOR

THE MILLION.

The Processes of Water-Cure Explained.

POPULAR ERRORS EXPOSED.

HYGIENIC AND DRUG-MEDICATION CONTRASTED; RULES FOR
BATHING, DIETING, EXERCISING, ETC.; RECIPES FOR
COOKING; DIRECTIONS FOR HOME-TREATMENT,
REMARKABLE CASES TO ILLUSTRATE, ETC.

BY

R. T. TRALL, M. D.,

AUTHOR OF "HYDROPATHIC ENCYCLOPEDIA," "FAMILY GYMNASIUM," "HYDRO-
PATHIC COOK-BOOK," "UTERINE DISEASES," ETC.

NEW YORK:
FOWLER & WELLS, PUBLISHERS,
753 BROADWAY.
1883.

CONTENTS.

Simple Fevers, Eruptive Fevers, Visceral Inflammations, Influenza, Asthma, Catarrh, Bowel Complaints, Spasmodic Diseases, Gout and Rheumatism, Consumption, Cachexies, Hemorrhage, Apoplexy, Palsy, Dyspepsia, Liver Complaint, Jaundice, Nervous Debility, Spinal Irritation, Neuralgia, Worms, Rashes and Eruptions, Burns and Scalds, Coughs and Colds, Dropsies, Asphyxia, Mismenstruation, Leucorrhea, Spermatorrhea, Venereal Diseases, Poisons.

WATER-CURE FOR THE MILLION

INTRODUCTION.

Hygienic medication—commonly called *Water-Cure, Hydropathy, Hygeopathy*, or more properly *Hygeio-Therapy*—is based on the fundamental principle that all curative virtue is inherent in the living organism; and that all that remedial agents can or should do, is to supply favorable conditions for the successful exertion of that power. Those conditions can never be supplied by the administration of drug-poisons, which are themselves incompatible with living structures, and which only cure (or rather *change*) one disease by producing another. They are only found in such materials and influences as the organism *uses* in its normal state; not in such things as it *rejects*. *Food, water, air light, temperature, exercise* and *rest, sleep, clothing, electricity, passional influences*, etc., are necessary and useful to, and usable by, the living system, in its state of health; and they constitute, also, its proper *materia medica* in all its conditions of disease.

So far from being a "one-ideaism"—as many charge, who regard the system as literally a *Water-cure*, and *cold* water at that—Hygienic medication embraces all the *useful* things in the world—every curative agent in the universe. It adopts whatever nature *appropriates*, and discards only what nature *rejects*. The "one-ideaism" is all on the other side. The term may well be retorted upon those whose remedial agents are, *whatever nature abhors and rebels against*, and whose only idea of a *medicine* is an animal, vegetable, or mineral *poison*.

The system of the healing art which I advocate and practice, not only repudiates all the remedies of the drug schools, but denies the philosophy on which their employment is predicated. It charges their practice with being *destructive*, and their theory with being *false*. It ignores all the fundamental premises of all drug-medical systems, and declares the truth to be the exact contrary of what they teach.

To illustrate: it is taught in all of their books and schools, that nature has provided remedies for diseases in the things *outside of the domain of organic life*. The truth is exactly the contrary. Nature nas provided *penalties*—and among them sickness—as the consequences of disobedience to organic law ; but she has not provided *remedies to do away the penalties !*

It is also taught, in all of their books and schools, that disease is an entity, a thing foreign to the living organism, and an enemy to the life-principle. The truth is exactly the contrary. Disease is the *life-principle itself at war with an enemy.* It is the defender and protector of the living organism. It is a process of purification. It is an effort to remove foreign and offensive materials from the system, and to repair the damages the vital machinery has sustained. It is *remedial effort.* Disease, therefore, is not a foe to be subdued, or "cured," or killed ; but a friendly office, to be directed and regulated. And every attempt to cure or subdue disease with drug-poisons, is nothing more nor less than a war on the human constitution.

It is further taught, in all the books and schools of the drug-systems, that medicines have specific relations to the various parts, organs, or structures of the living system ; that they possess an inherent power to "elect" or "select" the part or organ on which to make an impression ; and that, in virtue of this "special" "elective" or "selective" affinity, certain medicines act on the stomach, others on the bowels, others on the liver, others on the brain, others on the skin, others on the kidneys, etc. This absurd notion is the groundwork of the classification of the *materia medica* into emetics, cathartics, colagogues, narcotics and nervines, diaphoretics, diuretics, etc. Now the truth is exactly the contrary. So far from there being any such ability on the part of the dead, inert drug—any "special affinity" between a poison and living tissue—the relation between them is one of absolute and eternal antagonism. *The drugs do not act at all.* All the action is on the part of the living organism. And it ejects, rejects, casts out, expels, as best it can, by vomiting, purging, sweating diuresis, etc., these drug-poisons ; and the doctors have mistaken this warfare *against* their medicines for their action on the living system.

The treatment of diseases with drugs ever was, now is, and always must be, uncertain and dangerous experimentation. It never was and never can be reduced to reliable practical rules. An art is the application of the principles of a science to specific results. And a science is an arrangement of ascertained principles in their normal order and relations. These principles constitute the premises of the system which is made up of the science and the art. But in medicine according to the philosophy of all the drug schools, every one of its fundamental premises is false ; hence its science is false, and its practice must be false also.

On the contrary, the treatment of diseases with normal or Hygienic agencies and materials is founded on the demonstrable laws of physiology, and reducible to fixed and invariable rules of practice, and it affords the data for a true Medical Science and a successful Healing Art.

Wherever and by whomsoever this system is understood, it is adopted. Just so fast as people become thoroughly acquainted with it, they abandon all the systems of drug-medication. Thenceforth they have very little need of the physician, and never patronize the quack. They will not be killed by *regular*, nor imposed upon by irregular, physicians.

But an imperfect and superficial acquaintance with its fundamental principles causes many persons to err in the management of its agents and processes. The scarcity of properly educated Hygeio-Therapeutic physicians, and the incompetency and charlatanism of some who assume the title of Water-Cure doctors, have rendered it necessary, for the great majority who approve our system, to be their own physicians. Very few of them, however, have time, opportunity, and inclination to study our larger works; and for the benefit of such I have arranged this little tract. Attention to the rules and principles herein stated and briefly illustrated will, I am confident, enable any person of ordinary tact and judgment to manage all ordinary maladies successfully, and to avoid doing any very serious injury in any case.

HYGIENIC AND DRUG MEDICATION CONTRASTED.

All that I have said, shall say, or can say against drug-medication, and in favor of the Hygienic system, is more than confirmed by the standard authors and living teachers of the drug system. I will give a few specimens of their testimonies on these points. And first, let me introduce to the reader some of the most eminent of the living professors of our Medical Colleges:

"LOOK ON THIS PICTURE."

Said the venerable Professor Alex. H. Stevens, M.D., of the New York College of Physicians and Surgeons, in a recent lecture to the medical class: "The older physicians grow, the more skeptical they become of the virtues of medicine, and the more they are disposed to trust to the powers of nature." Again: "Notwithstanding all of our boasted improvements, patients suffer as much as they did forty years ago." And again: "The reason medicine has advanced so slowly, is because physicians have studied the writings of their predecessors, instead of nature."

The venerable Professor Jos. M. Smith, M.D., of the same school, testifies: "All medicines which enter the circulation, *poison the blood* in the same manner as do the poisons that produce disease." Again: "Drugs do not cure disease; disease is always cured by the *vis medicatrix naturæ.*" And again: "Digitalis has *hurried thousands to the grave.*" Dr. Hosack, formerly a Professor in this College, used to say that it derived its name from the fact that it *pointed the way to the grave.*" And yet again: "Prussic acid was once extensively used in the treatment of consumption, both in Europe and America; but its reputation is now lost. Thousands of patients were treated with it, but *not a case was benefited.* On the contrary, *hundreds were hurried to the grave.*"

Says Professor C. A. Gilman, M.D., of the same school: "Many of the chronic diseases of adults are caused by the *maltreatment* of infantile diseases." Again: "Blisters nearly always *produce death* when applied to children." Again: "I give mercury to children when I wish to *depress* the powers of life." And again: "The application of opium to the true skin of an infant is very likely to *produce death.*" And yet again: "A single drop of laudanum will often *destroy the life* of an infant." And once more: "Four grains of calomel will often *kill an adult.*" And, finally: "A mild mercurial course, and mildly *cutting a man's throat,* are synonymous terms."

Says Professor Alonzo Clark, M.D., of the same school: "From thirty to sixty grains of calomel have been given very young children for croup." Again: "Apoplectic patients, who are *not bled,* have double the chance to recover that those have who are bled." And again: "Physicians have learned that *more harm than good* has been done by the use of drugs in the treatment of measles, scarlatina, and other self-limited diseases." And yet again: "My experience is, that croup *can't well be cured;* at least, the success of treatment is very doubtful. A different mode of treatment is introduced yearly, to be succeeded by another the next year." Once more: "Ten thousand times ten thousand methods have been tried, *in vain,* to cure diabetes." Still another: "In their zeal to do good, physicians have done much harm. They have *hurried many to the grave* who would have recovered if left to nature." And, finally: "All of our curative agents are poisons; and, as a consequence, *every dose diminishes the patient's vitality.*"

Says Professor W. Parker, M.D., of the same school: "I have *no confidence* in gonorrheal specifics." Again: "Nearly all cases of urethral stricture are *caused* by strong injections." And again: "The usual treatment of syphilis, by mercury, causes atheromatous deposits in the coats of the arteries, *predisposing to apoplexy*." And yet again: "It must be confessed that the administration of remedies is conducted more in an *empiricial* than in a rational manner." Once more: "The pains of which patients with secondary and tertiary syphilis complain are not referable to the syphilitic poison, but to the *mercury* with which they have been drugged." And, finally: "Of all sciences, medicine is the most uncertain."

Says Professor E. H. Davis, M.D., of the New York Medical College: "Tablespoonful doses—480 grains—of calomel have been given in cholera." Again: "The *modus operandi* of medicines is still a very obscure subject. We know they operate, but exactly *how* they operate is entirely unknown." And again: "The vital effects of medicines are very little understood; it is a term used to *cover our ignorance*."

Says Professor E. R. Peaslee, M.D., of the same school: "The administration of powerful medicines is the most fruitful cause of derangements of the digestion." Again: "The giving of morphine, or other sedatives, to check the cough in consumption, is a *pernicious practice*."

Says Professor Horace Green, M. D., of the same school: "The confidence you have in medicine will be dissipated by experience in treating diseases." Again: "Cod-liver oil has *no curative power* in tuberculosis."

Says Professor H. G. Cox, M.D., of the same school: "There is much truth in the statement of Dr. Hughes Bennett, that blood-letting is *always injurious*, and *never necessary*, and I am inclined to think it entirely correct." Again: "Bleeding in pneumonia *doubles the mortality*." And again: "Calomel does *no good* in pneumonia." And yet again: "The *fewer remedies* you employ *in any disease*, the *better for your patient*." And once more: "Mercury is a sheet-anchor in fevers; but it is an anchor that *moors your patient to the grave*."

Says Professor B. F. Barker, M.D., of the same school: "The drugs which are administered for the cure of scarlet fever and measles, *kill far more than those diseases do*. I have recently given *no medicine* in their treatment, and have had excellent success." Again: "I have known several ladies become *habitual drunkards*, the primary cause being a taste for stimulants, which was acquired in consequence of alcoholic drink being administered to them as medi·

cine." And again: "I am inclined to think that mercury, given **as** an aplastic agent, does *far more harm than good.*" And yet again: " I incline to the belief that bleeding is *injurious* and *unnecessary.*" Once more: " There is, I am sorry to say, as much empiricism *in the medical profession* as out of it." And, finally: " Instead of investigating for themselves, medical authors have *copied the errors* of their predecessors, and have thus retarded the progress of medical science, and perpetuated error."

Says Professor J. W. Carson, M.D., of the same school: "It is easy to destroy the life of an infant. This you will find when you enter practice. You will find that a slight scratch of the pen, which dictates a little too much of a remedy, *will snuff out the infant's life;* and when you next visit your patient, you will find that the child which you left cheerful a few hours previously, is *stiff and cold.* Beware, then, how you use your remedies!" Again: " We do not know whether our patients recover because we give medicine, or because nature cures them. Perhaps *bread-pills* would cure as many as medicine."

Says Professor E. S. Carr, M.D., of the New York University Medical School: " All drugs are more or less adulterated; and as not more than one physician in a hundred has sufficient knowledge in chemistry to detect impurities, the physician seldom knows just how much of a remedy he is prescribing." Again: "Mercury, when administered in any form, is taken into the circulation, and carried to every tissue of the body. The effects of mercury are rot for a day, but *for all time.* It often lodges in the bones, occasionally causing pain *years after it is administered.* I have often detected metallic mercury in the bones of patients who had been treated with this *subtile poisonous agent.*"

Says Professor S. St. John, M.D., of the same school: " All medicines are *poisonous.*"

Says Professor A. Dean, LL.D., of the same school: " Mercury. when introduced into the system, *always acts as a poison.*"

Says Professor Martin Paine, M.D., of the same school: " Our remedial agents are themselves *morbific.*" Again: " Our medicines act upon the system in the same manner as do the *remote causes of disease.*" And again: " Drug medicines do but cure one disease by producing another."

Says Professor S. D. Gross, M.D., late of the New York University Medical School, now of the Louisville (Ky.) Medical College: " Of the essence of disease very little is known; indeed, nothing at all."

Such being the deliberate assertions, declarations, and confessions of those who advocate, teach, and practice the drug system, let us see next what they say of the system which we advocate, and which they oppose.

"AND NOW LOOK ON THIS."

Says Professor Parker: "As we place more confidence in nature, and less in preparations of the apothecary, *mortality diminishes*." Again: "Hygiene is of *far more value* in the treatment of disease than drugs." And again: "I wish the *materia medica* was in Guinea, and that you would study *materia alimentaria*." And yet again: "You are taught learnedly about *materia medica*, and but little about diet." Once more: "We will have *less mortality* when people eat to live." And, finally: "I have cured granulations of the eyes, in chronic conjunctivitis, by Hygienic treatment, after all kinds of drug applications had failed."

Says Professor Carson: "Water is the *best diaphoretic* we have." Again: "My preceptor used to give colored water to his patients; and it was noticed that those who took the water *recovered more rapidly* than those of another physician, who bled his patients."

Says Professor Clark: "Pure cold air is the *best tonic* the patient can take." Again: "Many different plans have been tried for the cure of consumption, but the result of all has been unsatisfactory. We are not acquainted with any agents that will cure consumption. *We must rely on Hygiene.*" And again: "*Cream is far better* for tubercular patients than cod-liver oil, or any other kind of oil." And yet again: "In scarlet fever you have nothing to *rely on* but the *vis medicatrix naturæ*." Once more: "A hundred different and unsuccessful plans have been tried for the cure of cholera. I think I shall leave my patients, hereafter, nearly entirely to nature; as I have seen patients abandoned to die and left to nature, recover, while patients who were treated died." And, finally: "A sponge-bath will often *do more to quiet* restless, feverish patients than an anodyne."

Says Professor Barker: "The more *simple* the treatment in infantile diseases, the *better the result*."

Says Professor Peaslee: "Water constitutes about eight tenths of the weight of the human body, and is its *most* indispensable constituent." Again: "Water is the only necessary—the only natural—drink."

Says Professor Gilman: "Every season has its fashionable remedy for consumption; but Hygienic treatment is of *far more value* than all drugs combined." Again: "Cold affusion is the *best antidote* for narcotic poisoning. If the medical profession were to learn and appreciate this fact [Why don't they learn it ?—R. T. T.], the number of deaths from

1*

narcotism would be diminished one half." And again : " The contin
ued application of cold water has more power to *prevent inflammation*
than any other remedy." And yet again: " The application of water
to the external surface of the abdomen, is of *great importance and
value* in the treatment of dysentery. I have also *cured* adults by this
means alone." Once more : " Water is equal in efficacy, as a diuretic,
to all other diuretics combined. Water is *the* thing that produces
diuresis ; all other means are subordinate." And, finally : " Water is
the *best febrifuge* we have."

Says Professor Smith : " The vapor of warm water is the *most
efficacious expectorant* we have." Again : " Abstinence from food is
one of the *most powerful antiphlogistic* means."

To the above testimonials against the drug system, and in favor of
the Hygienic, I will add the opinions of a few of the standard authors
of the Allopathic School :

LOOK ON THIS, ALSO.

" I have *no faith* whatever in medicine." Dr. BAILIE, of London.

" The medical practice of our day is, at the best, a most *uncertain*
and unsatisfactory system ; it has *neither philosophy nor common
sense* to commend it to confidence."

Professor EVANS, Fellow of the Royal College, London.

" Gentlemen, ninety-nine out of every hundred medical facts are
medical lies ; and medical doctrines are, for the most part, *stark,
staring nonsense.*" Professor GREGORY, of Edinburgh, Scotland.

" I am incessantly led to make an apology for the instability of
the theories and practice of physic. Those physicians generally
become the most eminent who have most thoroughly emancipated
themselves from the tyranny of the schools of medicine. Dissections
daily convince us of our *ignorance of disease,* and cause us to blush
at our prescriptions. What *mischiefs* have we not done under the
belief of *false facts* and *false theories !* We have assisted in *multi-
plying diseases ;* we have done more : we have *increased their
fatality.*" BENJAMIN RUSH, M.D.,
Formerly Professor in the first Medical College in Philadelphia.

" It can not be denied that the present system of medicine is a *burning shame* to its professors, if indeed a series of vague and uncertain
incongruities deserves to be called by that name. How rarely do our
medicines do good ! How often do they make our patients *really
worse !* I fearlessly assert that in most cases the sufferer would be
safer without a physician than with one. I have seen enough of the

mal-practice of my professional brethren to warrant the strong language I employ."

Dr. RAMAGE, Fellow of the Royal College, London.

" Assuredly the uncertain and most unsatisfactory art that we call medical science, is *no science at all*, but a jumble of inconsistent opinions; of conclusions hastily and often incorrectly drawn ; of facts misunderstood or perverted; of comparisons without analogy ; of hypotheses without reason, and theories not only useless, but *dangerous.*" *Dublin Medical Journal.*

" Some patients get well with the aid of medicine; more without it; and still more *in spite of it.*"

Sir JOHN FORBES, M.D., F.R.S., Physician to Queen Victoria.

" Thousands are annually *slaughtered* in the quiet sick-room. Governments should at once either banish medical men, and proscribe their *blundering art*, or they should adopt some better means to protect the lives of the people than at present prevail, when they look far less after the practice of this *dangerous profession*, and the *murders* committed in it, than after the lowest trades."

Dr. FRANK, an eminent European Author and Practitioner.

" Let us no longer wonder at the lamentable want of success which marks our practice, when there is scarcely a sound physiological principle among us. I hesitate not to declare, no matter how sorely I shall wound our vanity, that *so gross is our ignorance* of the real nature of the physiological disorder called disease, that it would, perhaps, be better to do nothing, and resign the complaint into the hands of nature, than to act as we are frequently compelled to do, without knowing the why and the wherefore of our conduct, at the obvious risk of *hastening the end of our patient.* "

M. MAGENDIE,
The eminent French Physiologist and Pathologist.

" I may observe that, of the whole number of fatal cases in infancy, a great proportion occur from the inappropriate or undue application of *exhausting remedies.*"

Dr. MARSHALL HALL, the distinguished English Physiologist.

" Our actual information or knowledge of disease does not increase in proportion to our experimental practice. Every dose of medicine given is a *blind experiment upon the vitality* of the patient."

Dr. BOSTOCK, author of the " History of Medicine."

" I wish not to detract from the exalted profession to which I have the honor to belong, and which includes many of my warmest and most valued friends; yet it can not answer to my conscience to withhold the acknowledgment of my firm belief, that the medical profession (with its prevailing mode of practice) is productive of *vastly more evil than good ;* and were it absolutely abolished, mankind would be *infinitely the gainer.*" FRANCIS COGGSWELL, M.D., of Boston.

" The science of medicine is a *barbarous jargon*, and the effects of our medicines on the human system in the highest degree *uncertain*, except, indeed, that they have *destroyed more lives* than war, pestilence, and famine combined." JOHN MASON GOOD, M.D., F.R.S.,

Author of " Book of Nature," "A System of Nosology," "Study of Medicine," etc.

" I declare, as my conscientious conviction, founded on long experience and reflection, that if there was not a single *physician, surgeon, man-midwife, chemist, apothecary, druggist,* nor *drug* on the face of the earth, there would be *less sickness* and *less mortality* than now prevail." JAMES JOHNSON, M.D., F.R.S.,

Editor of the *Medico-Chirurgical Review.*

These extracts, which might very easily be extended so as to fill a large volume, shall conclude with the following confession and declaration deliberately adopted and recorded by the members of the National Medical Convention, representing the *élite* of the profession of the United States, held in St. Louis, Mo., a few years ago :

" It is wholly incontestable that there exists a wide-spread dissatisfaction with what is called the regular or old allopathic system of medical practice. Multitudes of people in this country and in Europe express an utter want of confidence in physicians and their physic. The cause is evident: *erroneous theory*, and, springing from it, *injurious*, often—*very* often—FATAL PRACTICE ! Nothing will now subserve the absolute requisitions of an intelligent community but a medical doctrine grounded upon *right reason*, in harmony with and avouched by the *unerring laws of nature* and of the vital organism, and authenticated and confirmed by successful results."

And now, since the assembled wisdom of the medical profession of this country has condemned its own system " as erroneous in theory" and "fatal in practice," let us turn to the processes and appliances of the Hygeio-Therapeutic system.

BATHING.

1. WET-SHEET PACKING.—On a bed or mattress two or three com‑fortables or bed-quilts are spread; over them a pair of flannel blankets; and lastly, a wet sheet (rather coarse linen is best) wrung out lightly. The patient, undressed, lies down flat on the back, and is quickly enveloped in the sheet, blanket, and other bedding. The head must be well raised with pillows, and care must be taken to have the feet well wrapped. If the feet do not warm with the rest of the body, a jug of hot water should be applied; and if there is tendency to headache, several folds of a cold wet cloth should be laid over the forehead. The usual time for remaining in the pack is from forty to sixty minutes. It may be followed by the plunge, half-bath, rubbing wet sheet, or towel-wash, according to circumstances. The pack is not intended as a sweating process, as many suppose, though a moderate perspiration is not objectionable. A comfortable temperature of the surface is the desideratum, independent of more or less sweating, or none at all. When the patient warms up rapidly, thirty minutes or less will be long enough to remain enveloped; but when he becomes warm slowly and with difficulty, an hour, or more, is not too long. In some cases it is necessary to put hot bottles to the sides as well as to the feet. When the object is to cool a fever, the sheet should be allowed to retain more water, or if the skin is very hot, double sheets may be used. In chronic diseases, when the main object is to induce "reaction," or rather circulation, toward the surface, the sheet should be wrung more thoroughly, and the patient enveloped with a greater quantity of blankets, comfortables, or other bedding.

2. HALF-PACK.—This is the same as the preceding, with the exception that the neck and extremities are not covered by the wet sheet, which is applied merely to the trunk of the body, from the armpits to the hips. It is adapted to those whose circulation is too feeble for a full pack; it is also often employed as a preparation for the full pack.

3. HALF-BATH.—An oval or oblong tub is most convenient, though any vessel allowing a patient to sit down with the legs extended will answer. The water should cover the lower extremities and about half of the abdomen. While in the bath, the patient, if able, should rub the lower extremities, while the attendant rubs the chest, back, and abdomen.

4. HIP OR SITZ-BATH.—Any small-sized wash-tub will do for this, although tubs constructed with a straight back, and raised four or five inches from the floor, are much the most agreeable. The water

should just cover the hips and lower part of the abdomen. A blanket should be thrown over the patient, who will find it also useful to rub or knead the abdomen with the hand or fingers during the bath.

5. FOOT-BATH.—Any small vessel, as a pail, will answer. Usually the water should be about ankle-deep; but very delicate invalids, or extremely susceptible persons, should not have the water more than half an inch to one inch in depth. During the bath, the feet should be kept in gentle motion. Walking foot-baths are excellent in warm weather, where a cool stream can be found.

6. WET AND COLD FOOT-BATH.—Place the feet in water as warm as can be borne for five to ten minutes; then dip them for a moment in cold water, and wipe dry.

7. RUBBING WET-SHEET.—If the sheet is used *drippingly* wet, the patient stands in the tub; if wrung so as not to drip, it may be used on a carpet or in any place. The sheet is thrown around the body, which it completely envelops below the neck; the attendant rubs the body over the sheet (not with it), the patient exercising himself at the same time by rubbing in front.

8. PAIL-DOUCHE.—This means simply pouring water over the chest and shoulders from a pail.

9. STREAM-DOUCHE.—A stream of water may be applied to the part or parts affected, by pouring from a pitcher or other convenient vessel, held as high as possible; or a barrel or keg may be elevated for the purpose, having a tub of any desired size. The power will be proportional to the amount of water in the reservoir.

10. TOWEL OR SPONGE BATH.—Rubbing the whole surface with a coarse wet towel or sponge, followed by a dry sheet or towels, constitutes this process.

11. AFFUSION BATH.—This implies pouring water gently over the surface of the body. The patient may stand in a tub, or lie on the bed, the bedding being protected by a sheet of India-rubber or gutta-percha.

12. THE PLUNGE-BATH.—This is employed but little, except at the establishments. Those who have conveniences will often find it one of the best processes. Any tub or box holding water enough to allow the whole body to be immersed, with the limbs extended, answers the purpose. A very good plunge can be made of a large cask cut in two near the middle. It is a useful precaution to wet the head before taking this bath.

13. DROP-BATH.—A vessel, filled with *very cold* water, is furnished with a small aperture through which the water falls in drops. It is adapted to torpid muscles, paralytic limbs, tumors, etc. It should be followed by active friction.

14. THE SWEATING-PACK.—To produce perspiration, the patient is packed in the flannel blanket and other bedding, as mentioned in No. 1, omitting the wet sheet. Some persons will perspire in less than an hour; others require several hours. This is the severest of the Water-Cure processes, and, in fact, is very seldom called for. The warm, hot, or vapor-baths are, in most cases, preferable.

15. HEAD-BATH.—The patient lies extended on a rug or mattress, the head resting in a shallow basin or bowl, holding two or three inches of water, the shoulders being supported by a pillow. It is principally employed in chronic affections of the head, eyes, and ears. Wet cloths applied to the head, the " pouring-bath," and the " wet cap" are good substitutes.

16.—THE POURING HEAD-BATH.—The patient lies face downward, the head supported by an attendant, projecting over the side of the bed, which is protected by a sheet or blanket thrown around the patient's neck; a tub is placed under the head to catch the water, which is poured from a pitcher moderately, but steadily, for several minutes, or until the head is well cooled, the stream being principally applied to the temples and back part of the head. It is useful in severe cases of sick headache; in the early stage of violent choleras; in the early stages of fevers, when attended with great gastric irritation or biliary disturbance. In hysteria, apoplexy, delirium-tremens, nose-bleeding, inflammation of the brain, ophthalmia, otitis, etc., it has been employed with advantage.

17. FOUNTAIN, OR SPRAY-BATH.—This consists of a number of small streams of water directed to a particular part of the body. It may be regarded as a gentle douche or local shower. It is intended to excite action and promote absorption in the part or organ to which it is applied.

18. THE SHOWER-BATH.—This needs no description. It is not frequently used in Water-Cure, but is often very convenient. Those liable to a "rush of blood to the head," should not allow much of the shock of the stream upon the head. Feeble persons should never use this bath until prepared by other treatment. Placing the feet for a few minutes in warm water, before taking the shower, is a good preparatory measure for feeble persons. Standing in warm water, ankle deep, will materially lessen its shock on the brain and nervous system.

19. NASAL, MOUTH, AND EYE BATHS.—Drawing water gently up the nostrils and ejecting it by the mouth, holding water in the mouth, and holding the eyes open in water of a temperature suited to the case, are the processes indicated by these terms. They are useful in

relaxed and inflammatory affections of the mucous membranes and other structures of the parts.

20. ARM AND LEG BATHS.—The limbs may be held in any convenient vessel containing the requisite depth of water. These baths are useful in cases of fever sores, chronic ulcers, inflammatory affections of the joints, etc.

21. VAPOR-BATH.—Hot stones or bricks may be employed to gen erate vapor or steam. The patient may sit naked on an open-work chair, with blankets pinned around the neck; a small tub or a common tin-pan, holding a quart of water, is placed under the chair, and red-hot bricks or stones occasionally put in the vessel, so as to keep the vapor constantly rising from the surface of the water. Another very simple plan is this: Procure a one-gallon tin boiler, with a half-inch tin-pipe, having two or three joints and a single elbow. The boiler may be heated on any ordinary stove, grate, or furnace, and the pipe so attached to it as to convey the steam under the chair in which the patient sits, covered from the neck downward with blankets. It may be employed from ten to thirty minutes, according to the amount of vapor generated.

22. AIR-BATH.—The whole body is suddenly exposed to cool or cold air, or even to a strong current, and an excellent and invigorating process it is in many cases. There is no danger from it, provided the surface has a comfortable glow or temperature at the time, and the circulation is maintained by active exercise. Friction with the hand, a sheet, towel, or flesh-brush, is beneficial at the same time.

23. BANDAGES AND COMPRESSES.—These are wet cloths, applied to any weak, sore, hot, painful, or diseased part, and renewed so often as they become dry or very warm. The best surgeons have, in all ages, employed " water-dressings" alone in local wounds, injuries, and inflammations. They may be *warming* or *cooling* to the part, as they are covered, or not, with dry cloths.

21. THE WET-GIRDLE.—Three or four yards of crash toweling make a good one. One half of it is wet and applied around the abdomen, followed by the dry half to cover it. It should be wetted so often as it becomes dry. It is extensively employed in bilious and dyspeptic affections, female weaknesses, etc. When required to be worn for a long time, it should, after the first few weeks, be omitted occasionally, or worn only a part of each day, so that the skin over which it is applied will not become too tender. It should not be worn when it occasions permanent chilliness.

22. THE CHEST-WRAPPER.—This is made of coarse linen, to fit the trunk like an under-shirt, from the neck to the lower ribs; it is applied

so wet as possible without dripping, and covered by a similar dry wrapper, made of Canton or light woolen flannel. It requires renewing two or three times a day. It is useful in most cases of pneumonia, asthma, consumption, bronchitis, etc. The same precautions apply to its prolonged employment as mentioned under the head of the wet-girdle.

23. FOMENTATIONS.—These are employed for relaxing muscles, relieving spasms, griping, nervous headache, etc.. Any cloths wet in hot water and applied so warm as can be borne, generally answer the purpose; but flannel cloths dipped in hot water, and wrung nearly dry in another cloth or handkerchief, so as to steam the part moderately, are the most efficient sedatives. They are usually employed from five to fifteen minutes. They are useful in cases of severe constipation, colic, dysmenorrhea, hysteria, etc.

24. REFRIGERATION.—One part of common salt to two parts of snow or pounded ice makes a good freezing mixture. It is inclosed in a very thin cloth, and applied for a few minutes, until the requisite degree of congelation has taken place. It is useful in felons, styes, malignant tumors and ulcers, fever sores, cancers, and in some forms of neuralgia and rheumatism.

25. WET DRESS BATH.—This is a method of self-packing, enabling the patient to dispense with the services of an attendant. A linen sheet is fashioned into the form of a night-dress, with large sleeves, and after the bed is prepared, the dress can be wet and put on; the patient can then get into bed and wrap himself sufficiently to secure a comfortable reaction.

26. ELECTRO-CHEMICAL BATH.—A copper-lined bath-tub is necessary for this process. The patient is immersed in warm water up to the neck; one hand is brought in contact with the positive pole of a strong galvanic battery, the negative pole being in contact with the metallic lining of the tub. The water is usually acidulated, though in some cases alkalies are employed. From half a pint to a pint of nitric acid is put into the water for each bath. It should not be mixed with the water until the galvanic circuit is completed, either by having the patient in connection with the poles of the battery, or these in contact with the copper-lining of the bath-tub. The patient may remain in the bath from ten minutes to half an hour. This bath is very useful in a torpid condition of the skin with low circulation; in glandular obstructions; scrofulas, rheumatic and gouty affections; in chronic congestions of the liver, and to aid the elimination of mineral medicines and other poisons.

27. INJECTIONS.—These are warm or tepid, cool or cold. The former are used to quiet pain and produce free discharges; the latter

to check excessive evacuations and strengthen the bowels. For the former purpose so large a quantity should be used as the bowels can conveniently receive; and for the latter purpose only a small quantity—so much as can be conveniently retained. Small enemas of very cold water are highly serviceable in cases of piles, prolapsus, fissures, etc. The self-injecting syringe is the most convenient instrument. With a rectal, vaginal, and intra-uterine tube, it will answer all possible purposes, for old or young, male or female. These articles can all be furnished for $3.

28. GENERAL BATHING RULES.—Never bathe soon after eating. The most powerful baths should be taken when the stomach is most empty. No full bath should be taken less than three hours after a full meal. Great heat or profuse perspiration are no objections to going into cold water, provided the respiration is not disturbed, and the patient is not greatly fatigued or exhausted. The body should always be comfortably warm at the time of taking any cold bath. Exercise, friction, dry wrapping, or fire may be resorted to, according to circumstances. Very feeble persons should commence treatment with warm or tepid water, gradually lowering the temperature. All shocks, such as shower-baths, douches, plunges, etc., should be avoided by very feeble and irritable invalids; by consumptives in the second and later stages; by those who are liable to great local determinations, or congestions, as "rush of blood to the head," bleeding from the stomach or lungs, etc.; in displacements of the bowels or uterus; during the menstrual period of females; during any considerable crisis or critical effort; after the crisis or "turn" of any fever, or other acute disease; during the existence of any powerful emotion or excitement; soon after eating or copious drinking; in all cases attended with profuse discharges, as diarrhœa, cholera, diabetes, hemorrhages; during the suppurative stage of extensive abscesses or ulcers. The heat or feverishness which may attend any of the conditions or diseases above-named should always be abated by tepid affusions or spongings. It is dangerous to employ the wet-sheet pack, in prolonged or violent fevers, after the crisis or turn of the fever. Many errors have been committed in ignorance of this rule. Never eat immediately after bathing.

29. DURATION OF BATHS.—Many errors are committed by remaining in cold baths for too long a time. I have known cases in which dyspeptics and consumptives, at Water-Cure establishments, were kept in cold sitz-baths for two hours at a time, once or twice a day. This was intended as a derivative measure, but it worked very injuriously for the patients. Derivative baths, like all others, must be determined by the condition of the patient, not by the thermometer nor chro-

nometer. Sitz-baths of a mild temperature should seldom be prolonged beyond twenty minutes; more frequently ten to fifteen minutes are preferable. It is better to repeat all bathing appliances frequently, than to make violent impressions less frequently. Plunges, douches, and showers, if the water is cold or cool, should not ordinarily be continued more than a minute; when the temperature of the water is temperate, or tepid, they may be taken from five to ten minutes. Tepid half-baths should usually be taken from five to ten minutes. Sitz-baths, foot-baths, head-baths, arm and leg baths, etc., may vary from five to thirty minutes. But, as already intimated, regard must always be had to the temperature of the water and the circulation of the patient.

CRISES.

Those general disturbances of the system, transfers of morbid action, or aggravations of symptoms, constituting crises, do not occur so frequently nor with so much severity in home-practice as under the more thorough and systematic course at a water-cure. Nevertheless they do occasionally occur; and then all the patient has to do is to moderate the treatment in precise ratio to the violence of the crisis. Keep quiet and cool, taking no more exercise than is agreeable to the feelings, and *let Nature have her course.* After it is over, if the patient is not cured, the treatment may be resumed as before. In some few cases, as in mercurial diseases, gout and rheumatism, the crises may be so violent as to render some part of the body excessively sore and painful; or the whole body feverish, tender, and inflammatory. In these cases one or two full hot-baths, ten to twenty minutes, should be employed.

Crises usually take the form of diarrhea, feverishness, rashes, or boils. Should diarrhea be very severe, it may be soothed by warm hip-baths. Feverishness is relieved by quiet, or a warm bath at bedtime. When rashes or boils become troublesome under the application of wet cloths, these should be omitted until the skin heals. It is a common error with people, and with some Hydropathic physicians, that crises are always essential to a cure. Many cases of the worst kind recover without any critical disturbance whatever. Nor should the practitioner ever aim to produce a crisis. If a crisis appear spontaneously in course of the treatment, it indicates a favorable effort of the vital powers, and is always followed by an improvement. But if provoked by excessive bathing, or mal-treatment of any kind, it is more injurious than useful. I have known cases, repeatedly, in which the patients were "under crisis," as it was said, for several months—in one case for two years. Such cases can be cured, by judicious management, in half the time that they are kept "under crisis" by the crisis doctors.

ABRADED AND ULCERATED SURFACES.—The best application to parts where the skin is destroyed, as in ulcers, burns, scalds, rashes, small-pox, erysipelas, and various excoriations, is dry wheaten flour. It should fill the cavities and cover the surface completely so as to ex clude the atmospheric air. Applied to burns and scalds instantly, it will stop the pain and prevent vesication—a fact which all families will do well to remember.

TEMPERATURE.

So far as protection from the atmosphere is concerned, the general rule is, to keep the patient so cool as possible consistent with comfort. In cases of burns and scalds, when the surface is destroyed, the pain may be very much mitigated by keeping the temperature of the room so high as the patient can well bear.

In the application of water, for hygienic or for remedial purposes, the invariable rule to guide us is, the temperature and circulation of the patient. The warmer his surface the colder should be the water employed, and *vice versa*. The sensations of the patient should also be consulted. The more feeble and delicate the patient, and the more susceptible his feelings to the shock or impression of cold water or cold air, the more carefully should we regard his sensations, in the temperature of the baths prescribed. Mischief is frequently done in home-practice, by applying the water too cold. Very cold or very warm baths should be brief, precisely in the ratio of their temperature. Tepid baths may be more prolonged. Baths may be regarded as *very cold* when the temperature is 40° or below; *cold*, from 40° to 60°; *cool*, from 60° to 70°; *temperate*, from 70° to 75°; *tepid*, from 75° to 85°; *warm*, from 85° to 98°; *hot*, above 98°. Hot-baths range from 98° to 115°; vapor-baths from 98° to 125° For bathing infants and young children the temperature should ordinarily be from 72° to 85° The greatest error in home-treatment is in giving too many so'd baths

WATER-DRINKING.

Thirst is the general rule for water-drinking. Those who use a plain, unstimulating diet have little thirst, and require but little drink. It is injurious to load the stomach with a large quantity of water when nature does not demand it. As with food, all that can not be used is a burden which must be thrown off. The routine practice of drinking so many tumblers per day, as is advised at some water-cures, is very reprehensible. It is well to take a tumbler of water after the morning ablution, and at other times according to thirst. It is unnatural, and hence injurious, to drink at meals. Throughout the whole animal kingdom nature has intended the saliva to be the solvent of the food. If the food is well masticated and insalivated, it will never need any water to " wash it down." In acute diseases there is often extreme thirst; and here water-drinking may be indulged *ad libitum ;* but it is better to " take a little and often," than to take large draughts at long intervals. In many cases of low fevers, cholera, etc., warm water will allay thirst better than cold. Enemas of warm water will also check thirst very promptly.

Cool, but not very not very cold, water is the most natural drink. But it is always important to have the water pure. Hard and impure waters are a prolific source of affections of the liver and kidneys. For invalids it is of especial importance that all the water taken into the stomach be *soft* and *pure.* Artificial " mineral waters," and the saline, alkaline, ferruginous, sulphurous compounds of the " medicinal springs," are pernicious beverages for the sick or well. The drugs they contain are no better, and no different in effect, than the same drugs taken from the apothecary shop. Those Water-Cure physicians who *permit* their patients to use them may be justified in thus yielding to popular prejudice; but to *prescribe* them, argues strange ignorance of Hygiene, or perhaps a worse motive.

FOOD.

DIETETIC RULES.—As fruits and farinacea are the natural food of man, preference should always be given to a vegetarian diet, whenever it can be had properly prepared. Those who use animal food should never eat of it more than once a day ; and they should restrict themselves to the lean flesh of vegetarian animals.

Milk, and its products—butter and cheese—though favorite articles with many invalids, are in no sense physiological or natural food for adults. A large experience in this matter has convinced me that all invalids (except infants and young children) can do much better without them. Eggs, rare-boiled, may be placed in this category.

The best forms of animal food are beef and mutton, boiled or broiled.

Fish, and particularly shell-fish, are among the least nutritious and grossest kinds of animal food.

With regard to condiments of all kinds, salt, sugar, vinegar, pepper, spices, etc., the rule is, the less the better.

Salt is an indigestible mineral substance, and in no sense dietetical. This last is also true of vinegar.

The best seasonings are the saccharine and acid principles of vegetables and fruits, as sugar or syrup. lemon-juice, etc. But even these should be employed in moderation

Among the fruits particularly recommended to invalids are apples, grapes, pears, peaches, cherries, sweet oranges, tomatoes, prunes, berries in their season, squashes, and pumpkins.

Of the vegetables we may especially commend potatoes, beans, peas, parsneps, asparagus, spinach, green peas, and green corn. Those whose digestive powers are not much impaired, can partake, without detriment, of cabbage, carrots, turnips, and cucumbers.

Invalids, however, in addition to bread and fruit, had better use but one or two vegetables at one meal.

As a general rule, breakfast should consist of bread and fruit; dinner, of bread and fruit with vegetables ; and supper, of bread with a small allowance of fruit.

Those who use animal food should take it at the noon meal. The breakfast should be light, and supper very light. Those who do not use fruit at dinner, may use a greater proportion of vegetables.

Mushes, as wheaten grits, rice, hominy, corn meal, etc., may be used as a part of the bread-food, at breakfast or supper. But they should always be eaten with a hard cracker, dry crust, parched corn, or something that will insure due mastication and insalivation.

TIMES OF EATING.—I do not regard it as of very great importance whether we eat once, twice, or thrice a day, provided we are regular in our habits, and have a proper regard for the time between meals, and the quantity and variety of our viands. I have known patients do very well on a single meal a day. One of my patients—Miss E. M. Hurd, of Sparta, N. J.—who afterward became my student, and is now a physician and the wife of Dr. N. W. Fales, of California, lived on one meal a day for more than a year. When she commenced this plan she

was an emaciated dyspeptic, but became healthy and fleshy while ad-
hering to it. "I have heard Dr. E. P. Miller of New York, state in a
public meeting, that, being badly dyspeptic, and having read my work,
he adopted the vegetarian system, and for more than a year took only
one meal a day, in consequence of which he recovered good health.

I have known hundreds to improve rapidly in changing from three
meals a day to two. Probably the majority of invalids, and especially
those who are decidedly dyspeptic, will find it beneficial to eat but
twice. Those who take three meals a day should take breakfast from
6 to 7 A.M.; dinner from 12 M. to 1 P.M.; supper about 6 P.M. Those
who eat but twice should take breakfast at about 8 A.M., and the other
meal at about 3 P.M. Those who adopt the one-meal-a-day system,
should obviously *feast* about the middle of the day.

PREPARATION OF FOOD.—After all, the most difficult part of the
Hygienic system is the management of the dietary. Few persons know
anything about hydropathic cooking; and so perverted are the appetences of the masses, that to talk to them of physiological victuals is
very much like talking to a brandy-toper of the beauties of " clear cold
water," or to a tobacco-smoker of the virtues of a pure atmosphere.
Bread, which is, or should be, the staff of life, has, by the perversions
of flouring-mills and the bakers, become a prolific source of disease and
death. Much as the Health Reformers declaim against the abominations of pork, ham, sausages, and lard, as articles of human food, I am
of opinion that fine flour, in its various forms of bread, short-cake,
butter-biscuits, dough-nuts, puddings, and pastry, is quite as productive
of disease as are the grosser elements of the scavenger swine.

Nearly all the bread used in civilized society is made of fine or
uperfine flour, which is always obstructing and constipating, and
which is deficient in some of the most important elements of the
grain; and it is still further vitiated by fermentation, or by acids and
alkalies which are employed to render the bread light.

Pure and wholesome bread can have but three ingredients—meal,
water, and atmospheric air. The water is only useful in converting
the meal into dough; and the atmospheric air serves to expand its
particles so as to make light and tender bread. If properly managed,
bread can be made as light as ordinary loaf-bread with no other rising
than atmospheric air. To effect this, three essentials must be regarded. 1. The dough must be mixed to a proper consistence—neither
too stiff nor too soft. 2. The dough must be cut or rolled into cakes
or pieces so as to expose the greatest possible surface to the heat of
the oven. 3. The oven must have a brisk or quick fire. The hotter

the oven—provided it does not burn the dough—when the baking
process begins, the lighter will be the bread. The reason is this: The
heat, when sufficient, instantly forms a nearly impervious crust over
the dough, by which the air is retained, and, expanded by the heat of
the oven without being able to escape, separates the particles of the
dough, and thus renders the bread light.

If the meal is mixed with cold water instead of hot, and allowed to
stand and swell for several hours before baking, it will be nearly as
light as if mixed with hot water and baked at once.

As good bread may be regarded as the great regulator of the
patient's dietary, too much pains can not be taken with it. All
persons who undertake home-treatment should acquaint themselves
with the processes for making it. Bread made in the manner I am
about to explain can always be had fresh for each day or each meal,
and may be eaten so soon after cooked as sufficiently cooled. It
requires but a few minutes of time, and a supply can be made before
breakfast for the day. Or a supply can be made for several days. If
heated a few minutes, when two or three days old, it has the tenderness and flavor of freshly-made bread. It is still more tender if dipped
in cold water and then heated.

BREAD ROLLS.—Mix wheat-meal (Graham flour) with boiling water
quickly, by stirring rapidly with a stick or strong iron spoon to make
a rather soft dough ; as it cools knead it a little with the hands
make the dough into small thin cakes or rolls; prick them to prevent
blistering, and bake about twenty minutes in a hot oven. The baker
—an iron one is best—should be well dusted with dry meal to prevent
sticking.

The cakes should be one third of an inch in thickness, and one and
a half to two inches wide. When made into rolls (which is the best
form, as it exposes the largest surface to the heat and forms a thinner
and more tender crust), they should be about the length and thickness
of the finger.

When a large quantity is required, it is more convenient to make
them diamond-shaped. The dough is rolled out, cut in slips an inch
and a half or two inches wide, then cross-cut into diamond-shaped
cakes. The knife, roller, and board should be kept well covered with
dry meal.

Fine flour bread may be made light in the same way. But it must
be mixed with *cold* instead of *hot* water. It requires baking from
ten to fifteen minutes.

BATTER BREAD.—Mix wheat-meal with *cold* water to the consistence of ordinary batter for griddle cakes. Pour the batter into

any convenient baking-dish—the bottom of which should be covered with meal to prevent sticking—and bake in a quick oven. The batter may be half an inch thick, or so thin as it can be spread. The thinner it is the better, although if made very thin a large oven is required to bake much in quantity. For this reason the bread rolls are most convenient for families. An individual who makes bread only for number one, and who does not like the "muss" of working in dough, will find the batter-bread a very convenient article. I have, many a time, made it and had it cooking in a gas stove in less than two minutes from the time I commenced.

WHEAT-MEAL CRISPS.—Mix the meal with water, cold, warm, or hot, into a stiff dough; roll it out so thin as possible, and cut into small narrow pieces or strips, and bake in a quick oven. These are excellent for sour stomachs and irritable bowels.

WHEAT-MEAL CRACKERS.—These differ from the bread rolls in being very dry, hard, and brittle. In order to render them so, the dough is thoroughly kneaded, and then baked in a *brick* oven till the moisture is entirely evaporated. If kept dry they will retain their sweetness and rich flavor for several weeks. If kept in a very dry and very cool place they will remain good for several months. They are made a little smaller and a little thinner than the Boston cracker of the shops. All traveling invalids should supply themselves with these crackers. Fancher & Miller, No. 15 Laight Street, New York, manufacture them largely, and send them to order to any part of the country.

LOAF-BREAD.—Very good loaf-bread may be made of six parts of wheat-meal, two parts of corn-meal, and one part of mealy potatoes, mixed with boiling water, and baked in the ordinary way.

RYE-BREAD ROLLS.—Rye-meal (unbolted rye flour) may be made into bread rolls or batter-cakes in the same manner as for wheat-meal bread rolls. They are very light and delicious.

CORN-CAKE.—Wet coarse-ground Indian-meal with boiling water, roll it into a cake or cakes of half an inch in thickness, and bake in a hot oven. Some prefer this made with cold water, after the manner of the wheaten batter-bread. This is the old-fashioned and ever-to-be-admired "Jonathan-cake"—the "Johnny-cake" of "Down-East."

OAT-MEAL CAKES.—These may be made in the same manner as the wheaten bread rolls.

OAT-MEAL CRISPS.—Made in the same manner as the wheaten article. When these are thoroughly dried over a slow fire, they will, if kept in a dry place, remain good for months.

PUMPKIN BREAD.—Stewed and sifted pumpkin, or richly-flavored

2

winter squash, may be mixed with meal of any kind, and made into bread or cakes, in any of the ways already mentioned.

FRUIT BREAD.—Stewed apples, pears, peaches, pitted-cherries, black currants, or berries may be mixed with unbolted flour, and made into fruit bread. A little sugar added will convert the article into fruit cake.

SNOW BREAD.—When snow is plenty and clean, a light and beautiful article of bread can be made by adding to flour, or meal, two or three times its bulk of snow, and stirring them together with a strong spoon. It may be baked in the form of a cake or loaf an inch or two inches in thickness. The oven should be quite hot. It will bake in about twenty minutes. A little pulverized sugar, mixed with the flour or meal, will convert this bread into a very short and tender sweet-cake.

GRIDDLE CAKES.—Oat-meal, wheat-meal, or corn-meal may be made into a batter by mixing with cold water and baking on a soap-stone griddle. Some prefer hot water for oat-meal.

SQUASH CAKES.—Mix flour or meal with half its bulk of stewed squash, or West-Indian pumpkin; add milk sufficient to make a batter and cook on a griddle.

PASTRY.—Baker's pastry, and also "home-make pies," as ordinarily manufactured, are among the worst of dietetic abominations. But pastry can be made so as to be not only a luxurious but a wholesome article. Almost any kind of fruit, with a little sugar, and a crust of wheat-meal, or of rye and corn-meal, shortened with mealy potatoes, are all the materials required. Squash, pumpkin, and custard pies require the addition of milk.

PUDDINGS. — I regard all these dishes, even when made in the plainest manner possible, as things to be permitted rather than recommended to invalids. They are mushes, made thin, moistened, and baked. Indian-meal, hominy, rice, and wheaten grits are the best farinaceous articles for making puddings. Sago and barley are allowable. Stewed pumpkins, properly sweetened, with a small proportion of farina or corn-starch, with or without a little milk, makes a very simple and light dessert that some persons are very fond of.

MUSHES.—These dishes are preferable to puddings. Wheaten grits and hominy, well boiled, are the best mushes. When wheaten grits are coarse-ground they require boiling five or six hours. For an ordinary family they may be ground in a large-sized coffee-mill; and if ground so fine as convenient, they will cook in an hour and a half. Rye-meal, Indian-meal, and oat-meal make favorite mushes also.

Rice should be boiled fifteen to twenty minutes; avoid stirring it so as to break the kernels; turn off the water, and let it steam fifteen minutes. All mushes, when cold, may be cut into slices, and moderately browned in an oven, when they become so good as new—and even better.

GRUELS.—These are merely very thin mushes. They are properly regarded as "slop diet" for feeble invalids during convalescence after acute diseases, in cases of obstinate constipation, etc. Wheat-meal, corn-meal, rye-meal, and oat-meal are employed in gruel-making. About two tablespoonfuls of meal are mixed with a gill of *cold* water and the mixture is then stirred into a quart of boiling water, and boiled gently fifteen minutes. Rice gruel is useful in some cases of diarrhea.

PORRIDGES.—These are intermediate between mushes and gruels. Wheat-meal or oat-meal is usually employed. Half a pound of the meal to a little more than a quart of water is the usual proportion. They require boiling about twenty minutes. Raisins, pitted-cherries, black currants, or dried berries may be added if desired.

SOUPS.—Split-peas, beans, barley, and rice are employed in the pre-parations of hydropathic soups. One pint of split-peas, boiled for three hours, in three quarts of water, makes one of the best soups for vegetarians. Some add a trifle of sugar. Bean soup is made of similar proportions, and then boiled in a covered pan for four or five hours. Rice should be boiled until entirely soft. Barley should be soaked for several hours, and then boiled slowly in a covered pan for four or five hours. Tomato soup, made in the following manner, is a pleasant and wholesome dish : Scald and peel good ripe tomatoes ; stew them one hour, and strain through a coarse sieve ; stir in a little wheaten flour to give it body, and brown sugar in the proportion of a teaspoonful to a quart of soup ; boil five minutes. Okra, or gumbo, is a good addition to this and other soups.

BOILED GRAINS.—Wheat, rice, hulled corn, and samp boiled until the kernels are entirely soft but not broken nor dissolved, rank next to bread in wholesomeness. They may be eaten with syrup, sauce, ugar, milk or cream, or fruit.

APPLE DUMPLINGS.—Mix boiled mealy potatoes with flour into a dough ; roll it out to a little less than one fourth of an inch in thick-ness ; inclose in each dumpling a medium-sized apple, previously pared and cored, and boil or bake about an hour.

RICE APPLE PUDDING WITHOUT MILK.—Boil rice till nearly done, then stir in sliced tart apples, and cook about twenty minutes.

BOILED INDIAN PUDDING.—Wet coarse corn-meal with boiling

water, add a little sugar or molasses, tie the pudding in a bag, leaving room for it to swell, and boil three or four hours.

APPLE JONATHAN.—Fill a baking-dish two thirds full of sliced tart apples, sweeten to taste; mix wheat-meal with water and milk (a little cream will make the crust more tender) into a batter, and pour over the fruit until the dish is filled; bake until the crust is well browned.

RICH APPLE PUDDING.—Take equal quantities of very tart apples, well stewed and sweetened, and bread rolls or crackers, previously soaked soft in cold water; mix them and heat them thoroughly for a few minutes. Any tart fruit will answer in the above.

CRISPED POTATOES.—Boil good, sound mealy potatoes till a little. more than half cooked; then peel them, and bake in a hot oven till moderately browned.

POTATO SHORTENING.—Pare and boil good mealy potatoes, choosing those which are of an even size; pour off the water, and sift, while hot, through a wire sieve. An equal quantity added to flour makes the best shortening in the world for bread, pastry, cakes, etc. A little cream added makes a richer but less wholesome article.

ANIMAL FOODS.—As I never recommend animal food to invalids, although I sometimes tolerate the use of it in special cases, my remarks under this head may be very limited. Beef-steak, without butter or gravy, is perhaps the very best kind of flesh-food. Slightly corned beef, boiled until it is quite tender, is also admissible. Mutton chops, broiled, or the lean part of mutton, boiled, ranks next to fresh beef in wholesomeness. Eggs are not materially different in this respect. To cook them so hygienically as possible, pour boiling water on them, and let them remain on top of the stove, or near the fire, but not allowed to boil, for seven to ten minutes. Chicken, boiled or broiled, is next in order; and lastly, fish which are not oily, as cod, halibut, trout, perch, etc. Milk is rarely admissible. With dyspeptic, bilious, and rheumatic invalids it is decidedly objectionable. Nor should persons affected with constipated bowels, or profuse discharges of any kind, use it at all. Butter and cheese should be out of the question, although cream and curd may be allowed.

EXERCISE,

" Little and often," is the rule for most invalids. All exercises should begin and end moderately. The kinds of exercises should be as varied as possible, so as to bring into action all the muscles of the system. Long walks should be alternated with frequent runs and occasional rests. The most severe exercises should be taken in the early part of the day. Those who are able should take moderately active exercise before bathing (except in case of the morning bath taken on first rising), and still more active exercise immediately after each bath. A morning walk or ride before breakfast is always desirable. Calisthenic, gymnastic, and kinesipathic exercises and manipulations, except in their mildest forms, should only be taken when the stomach is nearly empty. Regularity is of great importance. Feeble invalids should commence all exercises very moderately, and gradually increase them in time and severity. Whenever much fatigued, rest or a change of exercise is advisable. Invalids should not get so fatigued as to be restless in consequence during the night, nor so much so that a night's rest will not remove all its disagreeable feelings. Those who can not go into the open air will derive great benefit from exercising in their rooms with the windows open. Dancing and the dumb-bells are among the most convenient in-door exercises. As exercise develops strength, the weakest muscles should be exercised the most; but if very weak, *passive* exercises should be principally employed for awhile, as rubbing, kneading, riding, sailing, etc. Invalids who do not react well after bathing, should be well rubbed over with a dry sheet by the hands of an attendant, and afterwards by the bare hands. Examples of all kinds of calisthenic and gymnastic exercises, illustrated with cuts, may be found in the author's "Family Gymnasium,"

VENTILATION.

All persons generally, and invalids particularly, should be very careful in having an abundant supply of pure air. This is very apt to be neglected in sleeping apartments. In sitting-rooms, warmed by the hot-air stove or furnace, the air is rapidly contaminated unless special attention is paid to ventilation. Indeed, no room is fit to sit nor sleep in unless there is some inlet for the fresh air, and an outlet for the impure air. In fevers and other acute diseases, fresh air should in all weathers be freely admitted into the sick room; and in putrid, infectious, and contagious disorders, as yellow fever, small-pox, etc., the supply should be abundant. Invalids will find it an excellent practice to *ventilate* the lungs each morning before breakfast, by half a dozen or more deep inspirations and prolonged expirations.

LIGHT.

The importance of light, as a remedial agent, is not sufficiently appreciated. Nearly all forms of disease are more severe and unmanageable in low, dark apartments. Many persons who live in elegant and expensively furnished houses so darken many of the rooms, in order to save the furniture, as to render the air in them very unwholesome. The scrofulous humors which prevail among those inhabitants of our cities who live in rear buildings and underground apartments, sufficiently attest the relation between sunshine and vitality. Invalids should seek the sunlight as do the flowers—care being taken to protect the head when the heat is excessive. Exposing the whole skin in a state of nudity, frequently, to the air, and even to the rays of the sun, is a very invigorating practice. For scrofulous persons this is particularly serviceable.

CLOTHING.

The physiological rule is, the less clothing the better, provided the body is kept comfortable. It should never be worn so tightly as to impede, in the least degree, the free motions of the body and limbs. Especially must it be loose and easy around the chest and hips, so as not to interfere with the action of the vital organs in respiration. Flannel garments next to the skin are objectionable. In very cold weather, thicker outside garments, or more of them, may be worn; but flannel under-shirts and drawers tend to make the skin weak and susceptible to colds. Invalids who are accustomed to them should leave them off in the spring or early part of summer, and so invigorate the skin by bathing, etc., that they will feel no necessity for them the ensuing winter.

SLEEP.

Invalids generally do not sleep enough. The importance of sound, quiet. and sufficient sleep can not be too highly estimated, as may be inferred from the physiological fact, that it is during sleep that the structures are repaired. The materials of nutrition are digested and elaborated during the day; but assimilation—the formation of tissue —only takes place during sleep, when the external senses are in repose. Literary persons require more sleep, other circumstances being equal, than those who pursue manual-labor occupations. If the brain is not duly replenished, early decay, dementation, or insanity will result. The rule for invalids is, to retire early, and remain so long in bed as they can sleep quietly. If their dietetic and other habits are correct, this plan will soon determine the amount of sleep which they require. Gross, indigestible, and stimulating food, heavy or late suppers, etc., necessitate a longer time in bed, for the reason that the sleep is less sound. And for the same reason, nervine and stimulating beverages, as tea and coffee, prevent sound and refreshing sleep, and thus wear out the brain and nervous system prematurely. Those who are inclined to be restless, vapory, or dreaming, during the night, should not take supper.

BEDS AND BEDDING.

All bedding should be so *hard*, and all bed-clothing should be so *light*, as a due regard to comfort will permit. Feather beds are exceedingly debilitating. Hair, grass, husk, chip, straw, etc., mattresses, made soft and elastic, are the proper materials to sleep on in warm weather. In winter a light cotton mattress may also be employed.

BODILY POSITIONS.

Avoid crooked bodily positions in walking, sitting, working, or sleeping. Always bend the body on the hip joints; never by crooking the trunk. Never lean forward while sitting so as to compress the stomach and lungs. Do not sleep on high pillows. Children are often injured and the spines distorted by this habit. Invalids who are so distorted, or so feeble that they can not keep the erect position in sitting but a few minutes at a time, should change their position frequently—walk, sit, and lie down, etc., so often as either position becomes painful.

NIGHT-WATCHING.

The usual custom and manner of watching with the sick is very reprehensible. If any persons in the world need quiet and undisturbed repose, it is those who are laboring under fevers and other acute diseases. But with a light burning in the room, and one or more persons sitting by, and reading, talking, or whispering, this is impossible. The room should be darkened, and the attendant should quietly sit or lie in the same or in an adjoining room, so as to be within call if anything is wanted. In an extreme case, the attendant can frequently step lightly to the bedside, to see if the patient is doing well; but all noise, and all light should be excluded, except on emergencies. It is a common practice with watchers to awaken the patient whenever he inclines to sleep *too soundly*. But this is unnecessary, because when the respiration becomes very laborious, the patient will awaken spontaneously. Under the drug-medical dispensation the custom is to stuff the patient, night and day, with victuals, drink, or medicines, every hour or oftener, so that any considerable repose is out of the question. But, fortunately for mankind, the Hygienic system regards sleep as more valuable than the whole of them.

FRICTION.

Friction, more or less active, is desirable after all ordinary baths, except in cases of fevers and acute inflammations. And in some cases of tumors, enlarged joints, and torpid muscles, active and prolonged rubbing, in promoting absorption and increasing the circulation, greatly assists the curative process. Many of the cures of these affections performed by specialists, in which cases thorough hand-rubbing is conjoined with the use of liniments, decoctions, and other medicamentums, are attributable mainly if not wholly to the friction employed. Wens, chronic swellings from sprains or bruises, etc., have been cured by the rubbing process.

ELECTRICITY.

There are two kinds of electrical force, mechanical and chemical. The former is the ordinary machine electricity, which operates mainly by producing shocks which agitate the motive fibers. It is quite analogous to friction in its effect, and is hence sometimes called friction-electricity. It is a convenient method for exercising, in many cases, particular sets of muscles, or exciting action in some particular organ or part; and to this extent is a useful remedial agent.

GALVANISM.

This is generated by alternate layers of metallic plates of opposite electrical natures. It is a powerful chemical agent, and as such is extensively employed in the arts. Its chemical action enables it to effect, to some extent, the decomposition of foreign and effete matters in the fluids and tissues of the living system, and thus favor their elimination. The galvanic current will often excite action and sensibility in semi-paralyzed muscles and nerves, and is sometimes successfully resorted to for the purpose of allaying rheumatic and neuralgic pains. The galvanic battery in connection with the warm bath in the form of the electro-chemical bath, is probably the most convenient and efficient method of employing the galvanic influence as a depurating agent.

MAGNETISM.

Whatever may be the intrinsic nature of the mysterious property known as animal magnetism, and whatever may be its relation to the life-principle, it is certainly capable, under certain circumstances, of exercising a powerful influence over the vital functions. The salutary effects of a cheerful disposition, a hopeful mind, and a healthy organism, upon the minds and bodies of invalids, are well known to physicians. Many persons are exceedingly susceptible to the influence of magnetism, while others can with great difficulty be impressed at all. In some cases it will quiet pain and restlessness, and produce sleep more effectually than opiates ; and in rare cases it can be made an efficient anesthetic agent to suspend sensibility, so that surgical operations can be performed without pain. Its laws, however, are not yet sufficiently understood to enable us to reduce its remedial applications to any very definite rules.

CLEANLINESS.

Few persons seem to have a proper idea of the full import of this term. Being next to godliness the term, cleanliness, implies perfect purity in all our mental and organic relations. Many persons who are exceedingly nice and fastidiously neat in their attentions to the external skin, and in the matters of apparel, bedding, rooms, furniture.

etc., are, notwithstanding, extremely heedless in regard to internal conditions and external surroundings. They will continually take into their stomachs and lungs such aliments and miasms as poison the blood and befoul the secretions; while they will permit the elements of contagion to accumulate to any extent in their cellars, yards, cess-pools, and out-buildings. I have known half a dozen members of a family to be prostrated with typhus fever, the chief cause being stagnant water and rotting vegetables in the cellar. Offal and garbage —dead and decomposing vegetable and animal matters of all kinds— in or around any dwelling, are a prolific source of disease. The hog-pen of many of our farmers causes more strange, putrid, and even fatal diseases than most persons suspect. I can hardly conceive of a fouler concentration of malignant and pestilent miasms than those which always emanate from a den of swine while undergoing the process of fattening. If folks will persist in keeping piggeries, they should be located so far from the dwelling-house that the abominable stench thereof will not be offensive to noses polite.

PRACTICAL HINTS FOR HOME-TREATMENT.

SIMPLE FEVERS.—When the heat is great and uniform over the whole surface, the wet-sheet pack is the best process, to be repeated so often as the heat increases. If the heat is moderate, tepid ablutions are sufficient. When the heat is unequal, apply warm applications to the extremities, and cold or cool ablutions wherever there is abnormal heat, aiming, always, to equalize the temperature. If the diathesis of the fever is very low, do not use the wet-sheet pack nor very cold water, except locally where there is disproportionate heat; but rely mainly on tepid ablutions, with such local warm or cold applications as the particular symptoms demand. In intermittent and remittent fevers, apply the wet-sheet pack only at the height of the hot stage. At the commencement of the cold stage, the full warm-bath, or the warm sitz and foot-bath are useful. Whenever the patient perspires profusely, and is quite warm, sponge the surface with tepid water; if the sweat is cold and clammy, rub the surface gently with warm soft flannel cloths. The bowels should be freely moved at the outset with injections of tepid water; and subsequently whenever there is trouble-some fullness or hardness of the bowels. Diarrhea may be allayed with warm sitz-baths and small enemas of cold water. Griping pains and local congestions may be relieved by fomentations, followed by cold wet compresses well covered with dry cloths. Retention or pression of urine requires alternate warm and cold applications, as does tympanitic affections of the abdomen.

Eruptive Fevers.—Small-pox, measles, scarlet fever, erysipelas, etc., are to be treated on the same general plan as simple fevers. When the throat is much affected in scarlet fever, cold wet cloths should be constantly applied. In the malignant form, commonly called "putrid sore throat," or "diptheria," it is sometimes necessary to use very cold water, or pounded ice, in order to arrest at once the process of disorganization. Bits of ice, or sips of iced-water, may be frequently taken into the mouth. In the malignant forms of small-pox and erysipelas the intense irritation of the surface may be allayed by the application of dry flour. This is good also to prevent pitting in small-pox. In measles, when the cough is tight and troublesome, the chest-wrapper should be applied.

Visceral Inflammations.—These affections, pathologically regarded, are fevers with a disproportionate local affection. So far as the fever is concerned, it is to be managed precisely on the plan recommended for simple fevers. The local affection requires something special, which is usually a cold wet cloth. In inflammation of the brain (brain fever), very cold water or ice should be applied to the head, with warm applications to the feet. Inflamed eyes should be covered lightly with a cloth wet in water of a temperature that feels most agreeable for the time. Inflamed ears should have *cold* treatment at first; but when the pain becomes of a throbbing kind, indicative of suppuration, warm-water fomentations should be applied. In inflammation of the tonsils (quinsy) of the larynx (laryngitis or throat-ail), and of the trachea (croup), cold wet cloths should be constantly applied around the throat, and often changed until the local heat and pain are entirely abated. In inflammation of the lungs (pneumonia), the chest-wrapper is appropriate. In inflammation of the liver (hepatitis), spleen (splenitis), stomach (gastritis), bowels (enteritis), kidneys (nephritis), bladder (cystitis), and uterus (metritis), the wet-girdle should be applied around the abdomen, or wet towels laid over the abdomen. In these cases, too, moderately cool hip-baths are useful.

Influenza.—This is a low fever with passive inflammation and great congestion of the lungs. The pain is not severe, but the breathing is very much oppressed. Keep the feet warm, and the head cool ; apply the chest-wrapper, wet with tepid water, and sponge the whole surface occasionally with tepid water.

Asthma.—A majority of cases are attributable to a morbid enlargement of the liver, or spleen, or both. The wet-girdle, frequent hip-baths are indicated. The pack and douche are proper for persons of robust constitutions. The diet should be very abstemious.

CATARRH.—This is a chronic inflammation of the mucous membrane of the nose and frontal sinuses. It is obstinate, and has its origin in a diseased stomach or liver. The dietary can not be too plain, and must be abstemious. Butter and milk are particularly objectionable. Hip and foot baths are always useful; a morning ablution, half-bath, pack-plunge, or douche may be taken, according to the vigor of the external circulation. The wet-girdle is generally advisable.

BOWEL COMPLAINTS.—Colics, choleras, diarrheas, and dysentery constitute what are commonly known as bowel complaints. When there is much heat in the abdomen, with tenderness, increased on pressure, several folds of cold wet cloths should be applied. If the sense of heat is trifling and the pain not increased on pressure, and if the pain is of the griping or aching rather than the acute or burning kind, warm applications or fomentations should be applied, and warm water given as drink. When there is nausea or retching, warm water should be drank freely until the distress is relieved or vomiting is induced. The bowels, in the outset, should be freely evacuated by means of tepid injections, after which small quantities of cool or cold water should be occasionally injected. When there is a sense of burning heat in the stomach, as in the spasmodic cholera, bits of ice may be frequently swallowed. In the latter stage of choleras the hot-bath, followed by tepid ablutions and persevering friction, should be resorted to. Ordinary diarrheas are relieved by the warm hip-bath. When dysentery is malignant with low typhoid fever, the warm-bath and fomentations are necessary, to be followed, if the pain and heat of the abdomen increase, by cold applications. When the tenesmus is very distressing, injections of tepid water and prolonged tepid hip-baths are necessary. The whole surface, in all of these complaints, should be packed, or bathed frequently with tepid, cool, or cold water, according to the temperature, as in the cases of fever and inflammations.

SPASMODIC DISEASES.—The convulsions of children are almost invariably caused by constipated bowels; and the principal remedy is, therefore, copious enemas to move the bowels freely. Epileptic fits are attributable, in most cases, to obstructions in some of the organs, hence the most important part of the remedial plan relates to the dietary and the action of the bowels. During the paroxysm little can be done except to keep the patient from injuring himself. During the intervals, ablutions, hip and foot baths are usually indicated. Hysteric spasms can often be arrested promptly by means of cold applications

to the head and fomentations to the abdomen. In those more formi-
dable manifestations of convulsive disease, tetanus and hydrophobia,
we have had as yet but little opportunity to test the efficacy of water-
treatment. I have, however, great faith in alternate warm and cold
bathing, and in the prolonged tepid half-bath. This plan is excellent
in cases of delirium tremens.

GOUT AND RHEUMATISM.—These diseases are essentially inflamma
tory affections of the joints with more or less constitutional feverishness. The febrile disturbance is to be treated according to its type
and diathesis, as in all other forms of fever. The affected joints
should be constantly covered with wet bandages, very frequently
renewed, and continued till the heat, swelling, and pain are entirely
abated. After the acute stage has subsided, the douche is useful.
There is no danger whatever that the external application of cold
water to gouty or rheumatic joints will cause the disease to "strike
in," and go to the heart, brain, or lungs. These metastases are always
the result of bleeding, colchicum, niter, mercury, antimony, or other
reducing agents and processes. The diet should in all cases be
abstemious. Rheumatic patients who have been severely salivated
can not bear very cold treatment; and gouty patients who have been
bled freely, should always be treated with water of a very mild
temperature.

CONSUMPTION.—In the incipient stages, provided the patient has
not been exhausted by prior diseases, as dyspepsia, hemoptysis,
spermatorrhea, mismensturation, repelled eruptions, etc., and has not
been bled nor drugged much, the wet-sheet pack, followed by a
moderate douche, is borne with advantage. In other cases the tepid
half-bath must be substituted. The chest-wrapper should be worn
constantly when there is much heat in and about the lungs. Hip and
foot baths are always useful as derivatives; and in the latter stages we
must depend on these with tepid ablutions, so far as bathing is concerned.
When hectic fever attends, so that the patient is chilly in the morning
and feverish in the latter part of the day, he should bathe only during
the hot stage. If troubled at night, the bedding should be very light,
and a tepid sponge-bath taken at bedtime. All exercises should
have special reference to expanding the chest so much as possible;
and the diet must be extremely simple and rather abstemious. A
little of the "hunger-cure" would be no disadvantage to most consumptives. If the lungs are greatly obstructed with tubercles or
abscesses, so that respiration is very much impeded, very little food
can be used, and more than this becomes an additional burden. It is
true that ninety-nine physicians of every hundred prescribe exactly

the contrary plan, and recommend their patients to *increase* the quantity of food as the respiratory function is diminished. But I think that the uniform result of their prescriptions—death—is presumptive evidence that their plan of treatment is exactly the contrary of what it should be.

CACHEXIES.—Scrofula, in its various forms of humors and tumors, glandular enlargements, white swelling, cutaneous eruptions, fever sores, rickets, lumbar abscess, hip-disease, otitis, ophthalmia, etc., as well as plethora, scurvy, elephantiasis, cancer, etc., require all the appliances of purification and invigoration that can be brought to bear upon the system. Plenty of pure air, abundant sunshine, and out-door exercises are to be allowed especial prominence in the remedial plan. The diet should be rigidly physiological. Bathing, as in all cases, must be governed by the temperature of the patient, the rule being to have all applications so cool as may be without being very disagreeable to the patient. Ulcers and swellings are to be covered with wet bandages. The dripping-sheet and half-bath are well adapted to a majority of cachectic patients. The electro-chemical baths are also useful. The air-bath is admirable in these cases. Fine flour and fermented bread should be excluded from the dietary. The majority of the food taken should be hard and solid, so as to secure thorough mastication. Wheat-meal crackers, parched corn, oat-meal crisps, and uncooked apples are to be specially commended to this class of invalids.

HEMORRHAGE.—Bleeding from the nose (epistaxis), stomach (hematemesis), lungs (hemoptysis), kidneys (hematuria), uterus (menorrhagia), and bowels (hemorrhoids), require cold applications to or near the part, a quiet recumbent posture, free exposure to cool air, occasional sips of cold or iced-water, and a very spare diet. The extremities should be kept warm, and the surface clothed according to its temperature.

APOPLEXY.—Cold cloths to the head, or the pouring head-bath, warm applications to the feet, tepid ablutions to the whole surface, and copious enemas to free the bowels, constitute the remedial plan. The head should be well raised.

PALSY.—Palsy of one side (hemiplegia), is connected more particularly with diseases of the liver and spleen. Palsy of the lower extremities (paraplegia) is generally the result of injuries to the spine, or of constipation and fecal accumulations; and palsy of a particular set of muscles (particular palsy) is almost always the result of mineral or narcotic poisons. The electro-chemical baths are more or less useful in all of these forms of paralysis. In a majority of cases the wet-sheet pack, warm, tepid, or cool, is useful. In the more feeble cases we must rely on tepid ablutions and friction. The dietary recommended for cachectic patients will apply to the paralytic.

DYSPEPSIA.—Plain solid food, water-drinking according to thirst, horseback-riding, climbing mountains, dancing the schottisch, with the morning ablution and half-bath, and a hip-bath once or twice a-day, are the things to be commended to the attention of dyspeptic invalids. If constipation of the bowels exist, a tepid enema should be taken every morning until they are disposed to act without it. Two meals a-day are better than more for the majority of dyspeptics. All greasy things should be avoided ; vinegar should not be used at all ; and sugar, except in very small quantities with fruit, is especially objectionable. Sour stomach and water-brash require a dry diet. When there is pain or heat after meals, the wet-girdle should be worn. The sense of "goneness," so often complained of, is best relieved by abdominal manipulations and the wet-girdle.

LIVER COMPLAINT.—Wear the wet-girdle during the night when the weather is cold, and during the day when it is warm. In other respects treat it as for dyspepsia.

JAUNDICE.—The electro-chemical baths are very serviceable. The tepid half-bath, with the dripping-sheet and the dry rubbing-sheet, are the other bathing processes most commonly indicated.

NERVOUS DEBILITY.—This is generally the combined result of dyspepsia, liver complaint, jaundice, and drug-medication. Sometimes it is caused by spermatorrhea, and occasionally by leucorrhea. A mild course of bathing, with gentle exercises, pleasant avocations, and a strict regimen, are the essentials of the restorative plan.

SPINAL IRRITATION.—This is also the result of the combination of circumstances just named. Treat it as for nervous debility.

NEURALGIA.—Generally the consequence of mineral or narcotic drugs. The electro-chemical baths, and warm, tepid, cool, or cold bathing, as either proves the most sedative in the particular case, constitute the leading measure of treatment. Sometimes very warm, and at other times very cold, water will relieve the pain.

WORMS.—Restrict the patient's diet to wheat-meal bread or crackers, hominy, parched corn, and uncooked fruit, avoiding all saccharine and greasy things, and the worms will not long molest the bowels.

RASHES AND ERUPTIONS.—These should never be "cured," or rather repelled, with ointments, astringents, irritants, sulphur, mercurials, etc., as the consequence is often disastrous and always injurious

A judicious plan of dieting and bathing will purify the blood, and then they will disappear.

BURNS AND SCALDS.—Instantly cover the part with dry flour. If the pain does not soon subside, apply cold wet cloths, gradually increasing the temperature as the inflammation subsides.

COUGHS AND COLDS.—Take a hot-bath at bedtime, and a wet-sheet pack in the morning; move the bowels with an enema, and fast for twenty-four hours. If inclined to chilliness, remain in a comfortably warm room, and keep the feet quite warm.

DROPSIES.—As with consumptive diseases, dropsical affections are generally easily cured in their incipient stages, and with difficulty afterward. When supervening on long-continued chronic diseases, a cure is almost impossible. Especial attention must be directed to the action of the skin. Packs, when the temperature will admit, the rubbing-sheet, and the dry-blanket pack, are the measures usually indicated.

ASPHYXIA.—Whether induced by non-respirable gases, drowning, or narcotics, the main indication is to inflate the lungs. Place the patient in the sitting position, pull the tongue forward so as to prevent the closure of the glottis, and imitate the natural respiratory efforts by alternately raising and depressing the arms, at the rate of fifteen times a minute. Gentle compression against the abdominal muscles, while the arms are being elevated, assists expiration. This plan should be persevered in for some time before abandoning the case as hopeless. When insensibility has been induced by narcotic drugs, anesthetic agents, or a shock of electricity, the pouring head-bath and the cold ablution are advisable.

MISMENSTRUATION.—In painful menstruation the wet-girdle, tepid hip-baths, hot and cold foot-baths, and alternate warm and tepid intra-uterine injections are proper. For pale, feeble, anemic patients, the warm sitz-baths, fomentations, and the full hot-bath are often necessary. Obstructed menses require frequent tepid hip-baths, the wet-girdle, and active exercises in the open air. Excessive menstruation requires quiet, cool hip-baths and an abstemious diet. In severe cases very cold water should be injected, or pieces of ice applied. Chlorotic females should have a daily ablution, and abundant exercise in the open air. They should regard sunshine as the very best kind of " blood-food."

LEUCORRHEA.—Frequent hip-baths and vaginal injections with water so cool as can be borne without disagreeable chilliness, and a plain abstemious diet, are the specialties of treatment.

SPERMATORRHEA.—A rigidly simple and abstemious diet, with moderately cool hip-baths two or three times a day, and strict attention to the general regimen, are essential.

VENEREAL DISEASES.—Gonorrhea and syphilis can always be promptly cured by judicious water-treatment. In secondary venereal affections the electro-chemical baths are very useful. Inflammations, ulcerations, swelling of the glands, etc., should be treated on the general plan applicable to such morbid conditions when resulting from other causes. When chancres exist, the surface should be destroyed by some powerful caustic to prevent the generation of infectious matter. Gleet requires warm local bathing at first, gradually reducing the temperature as the discharge subsides. In persons of gross habits and debilitated constitutions, the full warm-bath, followed oy the wet-sheet pack, is the best purifying process. The ordinary drug-treatment for this class of diseases is, taken altogether, vastly more injurious to the constitution than the diseases would be if left entirely to themselves. There is no truth whatever in the popular notion, that mercury is a "specific" or an "antidote" for venereal infection

POISONS.—In a strict sense, everything which is not food is poison. Drugs and medicines of all kinds, whether derived from the animal, mineral, or vegetable kingdom, are poisons, and nothing else. So are all simple elements. *Every chemical substance in the universe is a poison to the living organism.* So are many organic products, as tobacco, lobelia, henbane, opium, etc. All of the acid, alkaline, earthy, and mineral ingredients—sulphur, iron, iodine, etc.—which are found in "medicinal springs"—are so many poisons. The rule to determine whether a substance has a normal or abnormal relation to the living organism—whether it is a food or a poison—is simply this: If it is *usable* in the normal processes –if it is convertible into tissue— it is food; if not, it is abnormal and poisonous. The poisons more immediately dangerous to life are the strong acids and alkalies, as aqua-fortis, oil of vitriol, muriatic and oxalic acids, potash, etc.; the corrosive mineral salts and oxyds, as arsenic, tartar-emetic, corrosive sublimate, etc.; and the narcotics, as opium, prussic acid, strychnine, aconite, etc.

It is not generally known, and very few physicians seem to be aware of the fact, that calomel, when taken into the system, is very liable to be converted into *corrosive sublimate.* In this way an ordinary dose of calomel may produce fatal effects. Thousands are killed in this way, neither patient nor physician suspecting the cause of death. There are many substances in the system, resulting from the continual changes of the organic elements, which are capable of thus converting a mild preparation of mercury into one of the in tensest poisons known. Free chlorine will do this, and this is readily furnished by common salt. No person, therefore, who uses salt as a dietetic article, and who takes mercury in any form, can have any assurance that corrosive sublimate will not destroy his life. Many persons have been severely salivated, and others have died very suddenly and mysteriously, soon after taking very small doses of calomel, blue-pill, and other *mild preparations of mercury.* I respectfully commend these facts to the serious attention of the mercurial doctors, and to the solemn reflections of their patients.

The general remedial plan in all cases of poisoning is the stomach-pump, if at hand, or if not, free vomiting, induced by the swallowing of as much warm water as possible, and irritating the throat with a feather or the finger. Acids will neutralize the alkalies, and *vice versa;* but it seldom happens that these things are at hand. The effects of arsenic and corrosive sublimate may be to some extent neutralized by the administration of albumen or gluten; hence the white of egg, milk, and wheaten flour are useful. Acrid drugs, as cayenne pepper, phosphorous, alcohol, mustard, horse-radish, cloves, etc., excite inflammation. The nervines, as tea and coffee, and those narcotics which combine nervine and stimulating properties, as all forms of alcoholic beverages, tobacco, opium, camphor, etc., are fast undermining the stamina of human constitutions all over the civilized world, and threaten, at no distant day, either to exterminate the race, or to reduce all the nations of the earth to barbarism. The worst bane of our country is undoubtedly tobacco. Its use is rapidly increasing among the young men and boys of this land contaminating their instincts, depraving their passions, poisoning their life's blood, wasting their vitality, deteriorating their whole organism, checking their development, and rendering them gross, filthy, sensual, and imbecile. And the medical profession, I am sorry to say, teach and commend, by their theories, examples, and practices, the doctrines which lead directly and necessarily to liquor-drinking and tobacco-using. They mistake stimulation for nutrition; and under this delusion they are leading the world into the ways of drunkenness, debauchery, sensuality, and all their ruinous consequences. They teach that alcohol—and the same is equally true of tobacco, opium, tea, coffee, and all other poisons which possess nervine, or combine nervine with narcotic and stimulating properties—*sustains or supports vitality,* or imparts something to the system whose action or effect is a substitute for food; and on this false assumption they prescribe it for nearly all the maladies which flesh is heir to. It will be difficult, I apprehend, to bring the masses of the people up to the total-abstinence principle so long as their physicians, backed by the standard authorities on chemistry and physiology, teach this pernicious error. It is the clearest logical proposition in the world, that if alcohol possesses this vitalizing power, the temperance people are all in the wrong; and if the temperance folks are right in denouncing alcohol as a poison, the doctors are as certainly wrong in pronouncing it a "respiratory food," or a "supporter of vitality." If it is a poison, it can not support vitality in any sense nor under any circumstances. If it can impart or support vitality, or supply to the system any necessary element of nutrition, it is not a poison.

For a full discussion of this subject I refer the reader to a small work I have written entitled, "The Alcoholic Controversy."

POPULAR OBJECTIONS ANSWERED.

1. "Water-treatment is *too slow* for dangerous and violent diseases."

Answer. It is the *most speedy* method of curing *all diseases* in the known world.

2. "It is *too harsh* for feeble persons."

A. It is the *mildest* plan of treatment ever invented.

3. "It is troublesome, and too much like work."

A. Health is worth working for. It is very convenient to take medicine, and very easy to die. A few drops of prussic acid would kill an invalid in five minutes, but long years of toil might be required to restore him to health. But which would the wise man choose?

4. "Pale, weak, and bloodless invalids can not bear *cold* water."

A. Nor should they take it. Such persons need *warm* or tepid applications.

5. "It shocks the system and disturbs the circulation, thus conducing to *organic diseases of the heart.*"

A. Nonsense. If too cold or too severe processes are employed, the result will be internal congestion and debility. But all this is unnecessary.

6. "Cold applications to inflamed, gouty, and rheumatic joints tend to *drive the disease inward upon the vital organs.*"

A. Nonsense again. They are just the things to keep it on the surface. Gouty and rheumatic affections are never struck in upon the brain, heart, or lungs, except in persons who have been reduced by bleeding or poisoned with drugs.

7. "In skin diseases the application of cold water tends to *repel the bad humors* to the internal organs.

A. Not so. Humors of all kinds naturally tend to the surface, and cold applications increase such determination, whenever there is preternatural heat. When repelled from the surface, it is always by depleting processes or poisonous drugs.

8. "Some persons have tried the wet-sheet pack, shower-bath, etc., with manifest injury ; *they did not react.*"

A. Very true. But it was malpractice with them. Either the patients were not in condition for such appliances, or the practitioner who advised them did not understand his business.

9. "The dietary—mostly vegetable—is too *low and meagre* to suit all constitutions."

A. It is the *most nourishing* diet that can be found.

10. "You exclude tea, coffee, etc., which to many persons are a *necessity.*"

A. They are no more so than alcohol and tobacco are to others. We take away all stimulants for the reason that they do not give strength, but *waste* it.

11. "Persons who live according to your system until they get well, are obliged to *continue the system,* or they are liable to get sick again."

A. And so they should be. A reformed drunkard can remain sober no longer than he lets intoxicating drink alone. Our system does not propose to *avoid the penalties* or disobedience to nature's laws. It is predicated on *obedience* to them.

12. "It deprives persons of many good things they are *accustomed* to."

A. Habit is poor authority for what is good or bad. Our system prohibits nothing that is intrinsically good ; but it opposes all *false habits* and *morbid appetences*—everything, in short, which is itself a cause of disease.

13. "The great majority of *regular physicians oppose it.*"

A. Because it opposes them. Its universal adoption would be the ruin of the medical profession.

14. "Some Water-Cure physicians *give medicine ;* others pretend to give none. Who shall decide when doctors disagree?"

A. Refer to first principles. Our system is *Hygienic,* not *medicinal.* He who practices drug medication is not a *true* Water-Cure physician, no matter what his pretensions may be.

FOR GIRLS. A Special Physiology; or, Supplement to the Study of General Physiology. By Mrs. E. R. Shepherd. 12mo, extra cloth, price, $1.00.

The following notices of this work are from Representative people, and are a sufficient guarantee as to its nature and value.

"Jennie June" says: NEW YORK, *August* 8, 1882.

GENTLEMEN:—I have read "For Girls" with care, and feel personally obliged to the author for writing a book that is very much needed, and that mothers not only can, but ought to place in the hands of their daughters. Mrs. Shepherd has executed a difficult task with judgment and discretion. She has said many things which mothers find it difficult to say to their daughters, unless forced by some act or circumstances, which alas, may prove their warning comes too late. "For Girls" is free from the vices of most works of its kind, it is neither preachy nor didactic. It talks freely and familiarly with those it is written to benefit, and some of its counsels would be as well heeded by our boys, as our girls. Respectfully yours,

Mrs. J. C. CROLY.

Mrs. Caroline B. Winslow, M.D., of Washington, D. C., in an editorial in the *Alpha*, says: "It is a book we most heartily and unreservedly recommend to parents, guardians, and friends of young girls to put in the hands of their daughters and their wards. It fully supplies a long existing need, and completes the instruction ordinarily given in physiology in our high-schools and seminaries. This book is rendered more valuable and important, as it treats with perfect freedom, and in a wise, chaste, and dignified manner, subjects that are entirely neglected by most teachers of popular physiology. . . . . None but a woman with a crystalline intellect, and a pure loving heart, could have written this clean, thoughtful, and simply scientific description of our sexual system, and our moral obligation to study it thoroughly, and guard it from any impurity of thought or act, from injury through ignorance, abuse, or misuse. It has won our entire and hearty approval, and enlists us as a champion and friend, to do all in our power for its sale, not for the pecuniary compensation of its author, but more for the lasting good of our girls, who are to be the teachers, wives, mothers, and leaders, after we have laid aside our armor and have entered into rest."

Drs. S. W. & Mary Dodds, physicians, with a large practice in St. Louis, Mo., say: "The book 'For Girls,' which we have carefully examined, is a valuable work, much needed, and it is difficult to say whether the daughters or their mothers would be most benefited by a perusal of it. You will no doubt find ready sale for it, all the more, as there is hardly another book yet published that would take the place of it."

Mary Jewett Telford, of Denver, Colorado, says: "Mrs. Shepherd has earned the title of 'apostle to the girls.' No careful mother need hesitate to place this little book in her daughter's hands, and the probabilities are that she will herself learn some helpful lessons by reading it. While there is no attempt made to solve all the mysteries of being, what every girl ought to know of her own organism, and the care of what is so 'fearfully and wonderfully made,' is here treated in a manner at once practical, modest, sensible, and reverent."

The Phrenological Journal says: "A book designed for girls should be written by a woman to be perfect; it being understood as a matter of course that she possesses a thorough familiarity with the subject she discusses. The author of this book indicates an unusual acquaintance with the anatomy and physiology of the feminine organization, also a ready acquaintance with the other phases of social relationship belonging to woman in her every-day life; with a more than common discrimination in gleaning just such material from general professional experience as is best adapted to her purposes. The style of the book is clear, simply colloquial, and has nothing garish, prudish, or morbid about it. It is bright without being flippant in thought, agreeable reading without awakening anything of the sensual or exciting. It concerns the healthfulness and the well-being of the girls who are soon to become wives and mothers of the world. There is no doubt but what many of the seeds of diseases in women are sowed in girlhood, and therefore this book should be placed in the hands of every young woman, and of every mother of a daughter in the land."

Address **FOWLER & WELLS, Publishers, 753 Broadway, N. Y.**

WORKS FOR HOME IMPROVEMENT.

The Phrenological Journal

AND

SCIENCE OF HEALTH.

The Phrenological Journal and *Science of Health*, having been combined, is now published as one magazine with the above title, and covers the ground hitherto occupied by both as distinct publications.

The Science of Human Character, the Laws which govern the Physical Organism, and the Relations of Mental and Physical Health to External Conditions, are the grand themes which belong to the special province of this magazine.

PHRENOLOGY unfolds the relations of Mind and its physical instrumentalities; shows how the multifold diversities of human character and capacity are related to universal laws, and by a positive analysis of individual mentality ministers to individual usefulness, designating special aptitude, and indicating the methods by which mental and physical deficiencies may be remedied. As an agency in training the young, in correcting and reforming the vicious, and in controlling the insane, its value can not be estimated.

This combined magazine will contain practical articles on PHYSIOLOGY, DIET, EXERCISE, and the LAWS OF LIFE AND HEALTH ; Portraits, Sketches, and Biographies of the leading Men and Women of the World, besides much general and useful information on the leading topics of the day. It is intended to be the most interesting and instructive FAMILY MAGAZINE published.

TERMS.—Published monthly at $2 a year. Single numbers, 20 cents. AGENTS WANTED. Address

FOWLER & WELLS, Publishers,

753 Broadway, New York.

"Know Thyself."

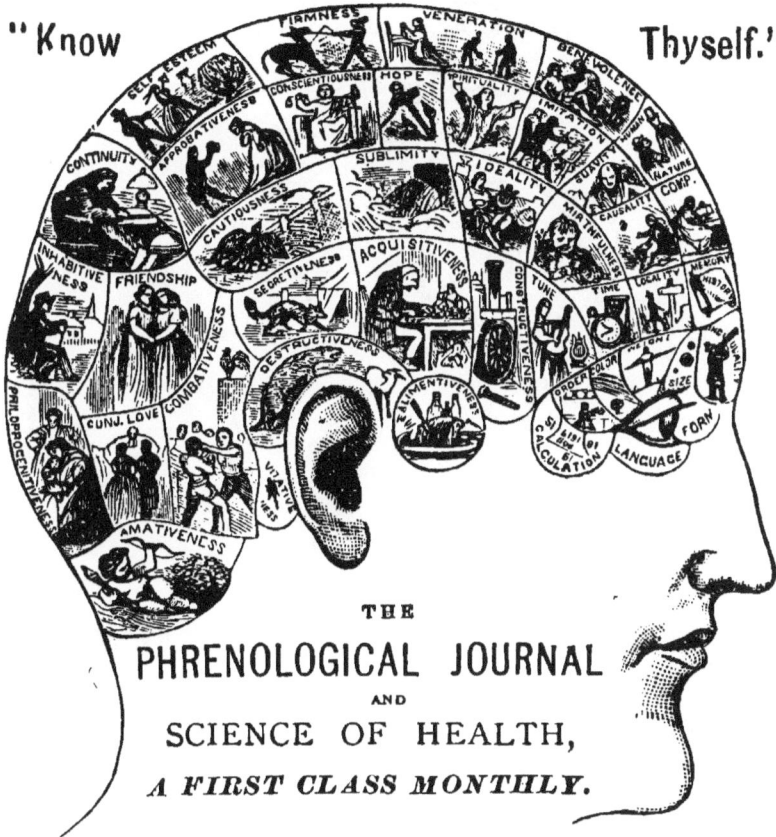

THE
PHRENOLOGICAL JOURNAL
AND
SCIENCE OF HEALTH,
A FIRST CLASS MONTHLY.

Specially Devoted to the "SCIENCE OF MAN." Contains PHRENOLOGY and PHYSIOGNOMY, with all the SIGNS of CHARACTER, and how to read them;" ETHNOLOGY, or the Natural History of Man in all his relations to Life; Practical Articles on PHYSIOLOGY, DIET, EXERCISE and the LAWS of LIFE and HEALTH. Portraits, Sketches and Biographies of the leading Men and Women of the World, are important features. Much general and useful information on the leading topics of the day is given. It is intended to be the most interesting and instructive PICTORIAL FAMILY MAGAZINE Published. Subscriptions may commence now.

Few works will better repay perusal in the family than this rich storehouse of instruction and entertainment.—*N. Y. Tribune.* It grows in Variety and Value. *Eve. Post.*

Terms.—A New Volume, the 76th commences with the Jan. Number. Published Monthly, in octavo form, at $2 a year, in advance. Sample numbers sent by first post, 20cts. Clubs of ten or more, $1.50 each per copy, and an extra copy to agent.

We are now offering the most liberal premiums ever given for clubs, for 1883. Inclose stamps for list. Address, FOWLER & WELLS, 753 Broadway, New York.

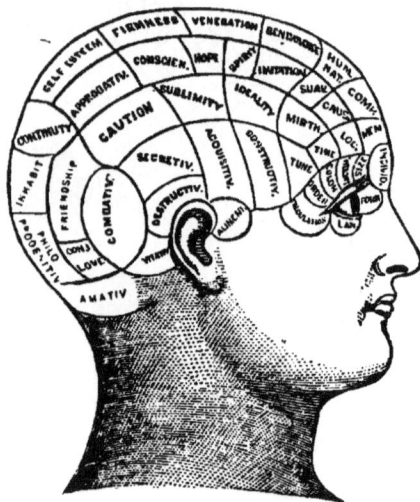

www.ingramcontent.com/pod-product-compliance
Lightning Source LLC
Chambersburg PA
CBHW030722110426
42739CB00030B/1175